MENTAL HEALTH MATTERS

I0486180

LEARN HOW TO IMPROVE YOUR SHORT-TERM MEMORY

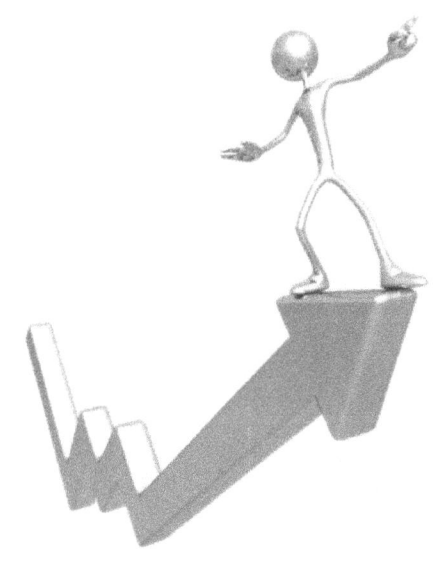

By Patricia A Carlisle

Introduction

I want to thank you and congratulate you for choosing the book, *"MENTAL HEALTH MATTERS: Learn How to Improve Your Short-Term Memory"*.

This book contains proven steps and strategies on how to improve your short-term memory.

Mental Health Matters (MHM), is a very important issue in human history. To make the subject clearer, we must start from the very beginning and origin of why and how mental health matters, and is associated to the brain that we inhale. Having mental stability or mental derailment is something that can determine whether an individual can really fit into the society. From the basic unit of life where a child is born, it is expected that children should develop under proper parental care, guidance, supervision, and the child should have a solid upbringing to begin with. The development of a child is indispensable, and cannot be over emphasize. Growing up in a healthy family, educational environmental, and proper nutritional or a balance diet including good psychological, physical, spiritual, exercise etc., will enable the child to develop properly and maintain a sustainable healthy mental state.

But, when the child is not given the right platform and enabling environment to grow properly, it will go a long way to hinder their mental growth and development. Many adolescent, and even adults are mentally retarded, just because the basic and necessary steps where not taken to address the important issues associated when Mental Health

Matters. From the above mentioned, the short term memory syndrome begins to originate and surface in life when the brain is not adequately develop from the cradle.

Thanks again for choosing this book, I hope you enjoy it!

ABOUT THE AUTHOR

Patricia A. Carlisle, MSW, CBT

Patricia Carlisle- a Cognitive Behavioral Therapist (CBT) gives out an expression of how important it is for an individual to take into consideration the concept of self-assessment to know what human, technical and conceptual skills they posses to perform or to achieve what they desire, or to deal with everyday life. However, every particular group of people has their own unique set of ideas, traditions and events including the frame of mind according to which people perform but there are many who faces problems and fail to maintain a healthy mind set affecting their behaviors and performance to those around them.

People like Patricia Carlisle are among those who have felt this urge of serving people and helping them out of their mental crisis towards a healthy life. She has experienced some close encounters in her personal life regarding mental health issues in her family and friends that has encouraged her to pursue this as her career.

Currently Patricia Carlisle is serving as a Certified On-Line Cognitive Behavioral Therapist with an extensive 15years of experience using Cognitive-Behavior Therapy Techniques. She envisions a world where everyone gets mental health treatment with no mental health stigma and to make it real she has already set up her own Holistic Measure Online Comprehensive Behavioral Healthcare Company after retiring from The Nord Center in The Partial Hospitalization Program (PHP) Dept for 5 years and Murtis H. Taylor Mental Health Center as a mental health counselor, psychological support technician and case manager for 10 years to emulsify her skills more professionally. Along with this, she has wrote down her passion as a clinician in 25 or more short books to help individuals and families get their life back, freeing them of the restraints of negative thinking, anxiety and depression by using different approaches. She is highly appreciated among her clients for her flexibility and professionalism of dealing with them graciously.

To reach her, make use of her direct website address: http://therapist2013.wix.com/e-therapy . As she is ready to inspire hope and contribute to health and well-being by providing the best online health care through comprehensive practice, education and research.

TABLE OF CONTENT

Chapter 1

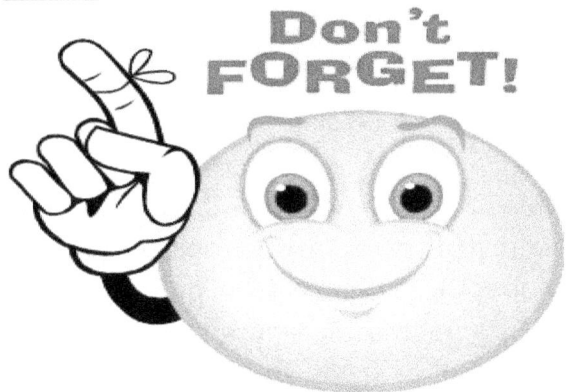

WHAT IS SHORT-TERM MEMORY

So what is Short-term memory? To be able to explain what short term memory is we shall examine the following instances. Short term memory is experienced when you are prone to forgetting the reasons or purpose of what you are doing intermittently, when you cannot remember what you just read from any book immediately after you finished reading it, when you tend to forget the names of those who are close to you, or familiar for instance, then it is crystal clear that you are facing what is referred to as short term memory loss challenges. The characteristic is very dangerous, and can really cost any person who is having such a problem expensive difficulties.

Typical problems associated with short term memory are instances when a student is given an assignment from school, and the student uncharacteristically forgets to do the assignment, and if this happens quite often to him or her, then the problem of short term memory can be traceable to the student.

When a employee forgets to carry out a basic task, or responsibility assigned to him, or a secretary frequently fails to deliver the message given to her to deliver to her boss, and she often forgets, then we can say the person has a short term memory.

These cases of forgetfulness can be very embarrassing and annoying, and may begin to cause a psychological effect on and individual. There are some people who put their lives under risk when they are prone to these symptoms of memory loss such as risking driving, not being aware of crossing a busy street, and risk being knocked down by onrushing vehicles, and so many other disadvantages that short term memory can cause.

Chapter 2

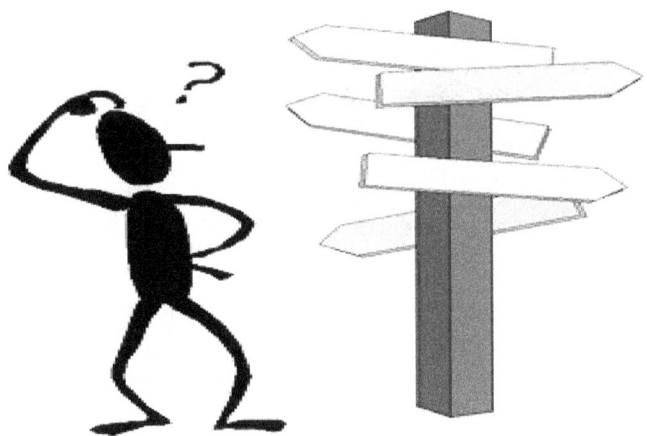

STAGES OF SHORT TERM MEMORY LOSS

In order for us to know how to improve short term memory, we will have to first of all learn the stages of memory available today. The study of psychology has been able to discover certain characteristic associated with the memory system of a person. The stages of these memory are categorize into three different sections namely, **THE SENSORY, THE SHORT TERM,** and **THE LONG TERM** stages of memory in the human system.

Indicated below is how the alignment of the memory links is inherent in the human system:

Sensory Input - Sensory Register - Short Term Memory (rehearsal) -Long Term   (FORGETTING)

As shown above: the normal travel of information begins from the organs of sensory perception through the motor neurons moving from the sensory organs to sensory register, and through the short term memory, and it finally gets to the long term memory where it is difficult to forget such information.

But when a person has the short term memory syndrome, the information when perceived from the sensory organs registers in the sensory register (where there are chances that some, or all of the information may not reach the short term memory), if however the information gets to the short term memory, and it makes a u-turn before getting to the long term memory, then it is established that the person has a short term memory.

Normally the sensory memory is majorly a sensory organ not lasting long, but only a few seconds, and is only meant for immediate perception. It basically functions as a photographical organ that captures images, or sound, or other forms of sensational activities; they are carried out by the sensory input memory. Often times, the perception received move swiftly from the sensory memory to the short term memory. The short term memory therefore act as a filtering interface only holding information briefly, hence, when information is processed in this platform it tends to remain there, and may further go into oblivion before transmitting, or may not get to the long term memory.

The long term memory is where the information can be held for a longer period of time is stored, and the likelihood to lose such information is very limited.

The Long Term Memory is the best memory, because of its ability to store retentive and valuable information. Besides, the long term memory has immense capabilities of storing information for a very long time, and the volume of information is always very high, and it can be stored there permanently. These special features of keeping information for a very long and extensive period of time indefinitely, characterize the long term memory as a superior memory. The long term memory can be compared to a computer hard drive, where information can be stored for decades without loss.

These are the different stages and phases showing how the brains functions. However, to actually determine the functionalities of the brain, scientist have only come up with stages of performance of the brain popularly referred to as "the Think Memory". The study of the brain is a continuous process, and there are bound to be improvement, and new discoveries as witnessed in many years past. Man's memory and brain capabilities seem to be advanced more than earlier men, the unique sophisticated and technological advancement has proved that man's memory is advancing everyday, and so new models of the memory models/structures and functionalities will likely be discovered in the nearest future.

The short term memory therefore, has been represented pictorially, but let us looks at it in deeper perspective. The short term memory is where little quantity, or tiny information are normally stored for about 15 – 30 seconds. The short term memory is not the part of the brain that is large, or engaging in large processes in the brain. Rather, short term memory utilizes small abilities such as temporarily memorizing a few set of numbers like phone number, account number, little comments, quotes, or conversation etc.

Just like recording information of a pad, the categories of information it receives quickly disappears, it is not stored, unless series of efforts are made to keep count, or recording the information immediately. The short term memory is also unique in a special way to the extent that you can utilize it to filter information, that is, decide on the necessary information that is worthy of storage, or information that needs to be discarded. Therefore, the ability of the short memory to select information and details that are necessary from the unnecessary information enables your brain to keep it from being overwhelmed by the huge daily information it receives every second of the day.

Chapter 3

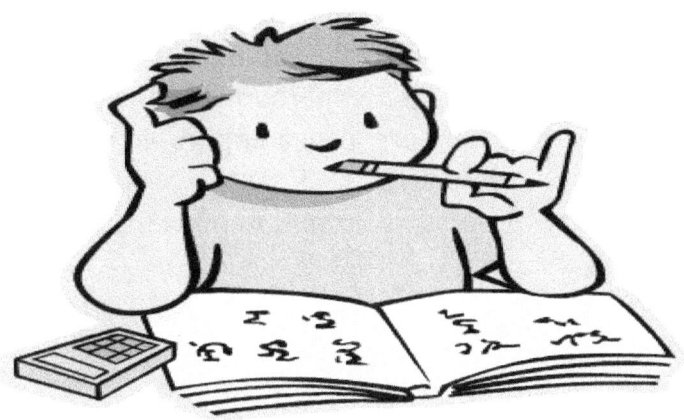

THE CAPACITY OF THE SHORT-TERM MEMORY

Previously, scientist always considered that the short term memory is capable of storing information up to seven pieces concurrently. But subsequent discoveries has disputed the fact that the short term memory may not be able to process seven pieces of information at the same time simultaneously, and scientists have now proposed that the considerable number of information that short term memory is capable of accommodating is four pieces of information at a time.

Some people also erroneously misinterpret short term memory loss, or equate it to be a temporary problem. But temporary memory loss like the one cause by headaches, transient memory losses, short term memory loss due to injury are not actually the same as Short-Term Memory problems. Therefore, short term memory loss is unconnected to how long you have it, rather it is what stage of the memory, that is, and sensory, short term and long term that is being affected at a particular point in time.

The working memory

The working memory is almost the same as short term memory; the term is used interchangeable with short-term memory by brain scientist. The method administered in improving the short term memory is also applicable to that of the working memory. Some scientist however proposes that the working memory process information more accurately than the short term memory.

Chapter 4

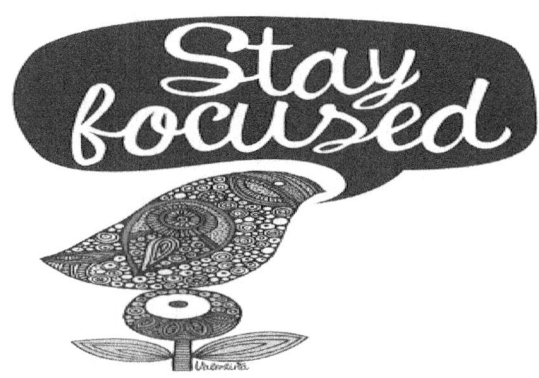

HOW TO IMPROVE YOUR SHORT-TERM MEMORY

Now that we have developed adequate knowledge about short term memory we shall now look at ways to improve your short-memory. It is interesting to note that short term memory can be very disappointing, frustrating, and embarrassing most of the time. You want to give permanent solution to the problem, how then can you go about it?

Pay attention and be Focus

The ability to pay attention to every matter or details that you come across every time will enable you to have the ability to improve your short term memory into a sharp memory. You can do this by interacting with the information you receive, try and give it a human face, and see it as something that needs your maximum attention, then you can begin to improve your short-term memory.

Carry out some Mental Exercises, and do one thing at a time

It will be very difficult for the brain to remember all the information that passes through it. Therefore, the brain has to pick some information, and discard the others. Most of the time, it's the necessary information that needs to be processed so go for relevant information. Try as much as possible to avoid distractions, because distraction is one of the reasons why people lose focus on what they are doing, and this often leads to mistakes sometimes the mistakes can be very costly and detrimental. If you lose focus while being distracted, you can end up being electrocuted while handling some electricity devices, data loss can take place, and if you are a doctor you may likely forget a surgical pin in the body of a patient while carrying out surgery, it is possible.

Full concentration: You may need to totally concentrate on what you are doing, do not worry about previous problems, or what you experienced in the past, do not worry about the challenges that you have all the time. Because worry will always take the better part of your thinking, and will definitely affect what you are doing. Your ability to develop a high level of concentration will further enhance your capabilities when it comes to learning and grasping new information.

Making use of Repeated Statements: What are repeated statements; these are statements made repeatedly in order not to forget. It involves saying words that you need to remember severally, and by doing so the chances that you will forget the words are slim.

Try Chunking: What is chunking? Chunking is the system involved in breaking information into bits in order to enhance the memorization of the subjects, or topics associated with the information that you intend to gather. If you form the habit of practicing breaking information into bits while you try to memorize them, surely with extension of time you will be able to improve on your short term memory. This is one of the most effective means of improving on the short term memory.

We shall quickly do some little demonstration, now, take a look at the number 345622445 it might not be that easy to be able to memorize this number for too long. But when you break it into the following lineal such as: 346-622-445. This is a very quick and easy way to grasp the numbers without a problem. Such scenarios will enhance and improve your short term memory.

Writing down information: Writing down information that needs to be remembered on a note pad is a very quick and easy way to improve your short term memory. If you forget the piece of information, you can always make references to it by revisiting your note pad, and get the information back to your memory. This is another basic way of improving your short term memory. Because as we explained earlier, the short term memory is a region of the brain that will always tend to forget things easily.

Take a trip: You can also improve your short term memory by deciding to go on a trip; it could be a short distance and less stressful trip. Do not stress yourself in the process, or else the feeling of frustration will begin to set in. Slow and steady wins the race. So make that little, memorable and enjoyable trip pleasurable to the extent that remembering things will be easy for you. So, while taking the trip try, and put into practice what memorable events that took place, and imagination of what transpired will help improve your short term memory. Also you can visualize the images of landscapes, and the natural environment which creates a form of resort, or relaxation of the mind.

Chapter 5

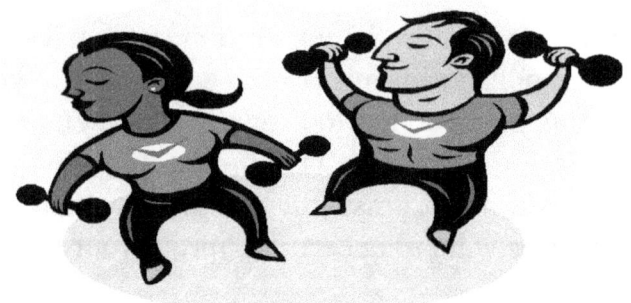

ADAPTING A BRAIN HEALTHY LIFESTYLE

There are some foods or meals that will not help the brain to develop adequately, hence, there is the need to develop a lifestyle that will make sure that your brain is advancing, or developing in the right direction. Do not expect to have an improved memory when all you care about or do is taking drugs, having relationship breakups, smoking marijuana, and doing things that will continue to affect the brain negatively.

Everything in life needs maintenance, your devices, your machines, cars, generators plants, even the garden that you are living in, or environment all needs someone to take care of it. If we do not take care of our equipment, then we should be ready for a breakdown of the machines, or they might just stop working. The same scenario is applicable to our body system, and especially the brain. So when we are talking about adopting a system that will improve the short term memory through a healthy life style, definitely it is not out of place.

Some other factors that are necessary to improve the short term memory is by imbibing a healthy eating habit by going for the natural food, avoid processed foods, and excessive sugar content will suffice for a better healthy eating habit. Also fresh vegetables, and fresh farm products will also be adequate. There is also the need to take adequate brain supplements this can be obtained from the Wellness Practitioners.

A lot of exercise, enough sleep will assist in maintaining a balance mental physique, and psychological balance. Being happy and doing stress free activity is also very important because stress is a very dangerous phenomenon that affects, and is capable of destroying brain cells.

Some Underlying Health Conditions that affect the improvement of Short Term memory include: high blood pressure, cancer, diabetes, depression, thyroid disorders, fibromyalgia etc.; these health problems are critical to the extent that it affects the general thinking, and functioning of the psychological disposition of the brain.

Hence, it is very necessary for an individual suffering from these health matters to visit the specialist, or doctor for a treatment for this first, before attempting to improve on his or her short term memory. For instance, a person who has diabetes will need to checkmate his eating habit when he is under the watch of a doctor who placed him or her on a diet that needs to be adhered if the person wants to be alive, and not put his or her health at risk.

So if your case is that of underlying health situation constituting the reasons why you have short term memory losses, then the best thing to do is to consult your doctor. This is the right step in the right direction to improving your short term memory.

Chapter 6

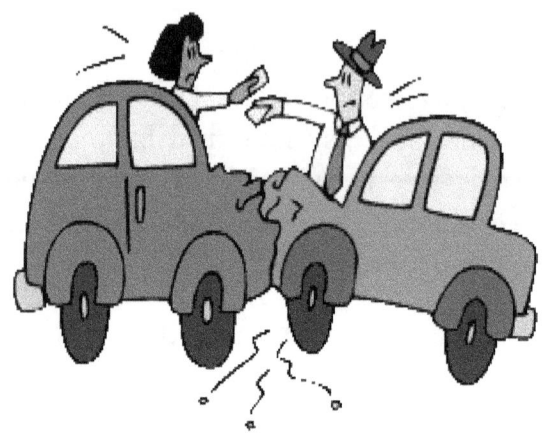

WHAT HINDER SHORT-TERM MEMORY DEVELOPMENT

We cannot discuss this topic without mentioning some unfortunate circumstances that can hinder short term memory development; some medical treatment can cause short term memory from improving e.g. Brain surgery, severe head injuries occurring as a result of fatal accidents, migraine, and taking sleeping pills, drugs administered for the purpose of lowering the cholesterol has contribute adversely to the improvement of the short term memory. Hence, taking drugs sometimes can be dangerous especially when the drugs have the possibilities of a side effect.

Therefore, when you purchase a drug always make sure it is the right prescription, and do not engage in self medication, a lot of people today are always making use of self medication to treat some ailments, or improve their health, this is very dangerous, so in order not to engage in self medication and harming yourself make sure you always seek expert advice on health matters. And, while you are taking medication as directed by the physician, always make sure you ask questions about the side effects of such drugs to be able to determine if it is a drug that will affect your short term memory.

You also need to do a lot more of exercise and rest, when you do exercise do it with a relaxed mind free of worries and frustration, listen to cool music, and also have a great sleep that will enable you to refresh your memory. Keep up with the routine repeatedly, and definitely you are bound to have successfully improved short term memory.

<u>Conclusion</u>

Thank you again for choosing this book!

I hope this book was able to help you find ways to strengthen your short term memory.

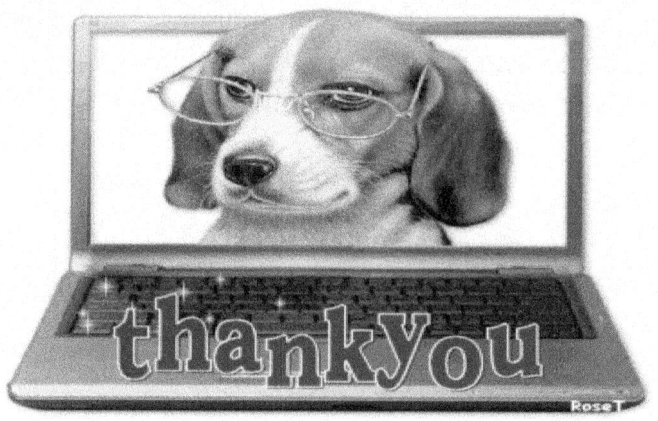

Finally, if you enjoyed this book, would you be kind enough to leave a review for this book on Amazon? It'd be greatly appreciated!

Thank you and good luck!

Preview Of 'MENTAL HEALTH AWARENESS: what You Need to Know about Mental Illness'
Chapter 1

WHAT CAUSES MENTAL ILLNESS

Although the exact cause of most mental illnesses is not known, it is becoming clear through research that many of these conditions are caused by a combination of genetic, biological, psychological, and environmental factors not personal weakness or a character defect and recovery from a mental illness is not simply a matter of will and self-discipline.

Heredity (genetics)

Many mental illnesses ruin families, suggesting they may be passed on from parents or children through genes. Genes contain instructions for the function of each cell in the body and are responsible for how we look act, think, etc. However, just because your mother or father may have or had a mental illness doesn't mean you will have one. Hereditary just means that you are more likely to get the condition than if you didn't have any affected family member. Experts believe that many mental conditions are linked to problems in multiple genes not just one, as with many diseases, which is why a person inherits a susceptibility to a mental disorder but doesn't always develop the condition. The disorder itself occurs from the interaction of these genes and other factors such as psychological trauma and environmental stressors which can influence, or trigger, the illness in a person who has inherited a susceptibility to it.

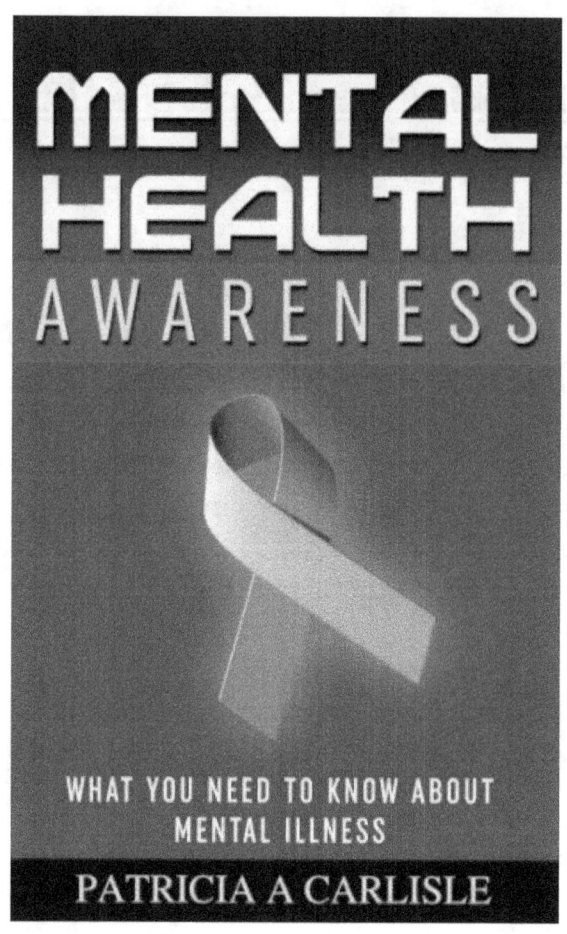

MENTAL HEALTH AWARENESS: What You Need to Know about Mental Illness.

CHECK OUT MY OTHER BOOKS

Below you'll find some of my other popular books that are popular on Amazon and Kindle as well. Alternatively, you can visit my author page on Amazon to see other work done by me. (https://amazon.com/author/patriciacarlisle)

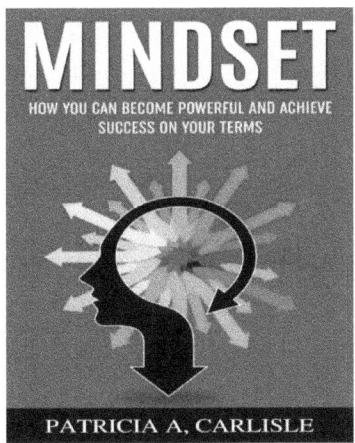

Mindset: How you can become powerful and achieve success on your terms.

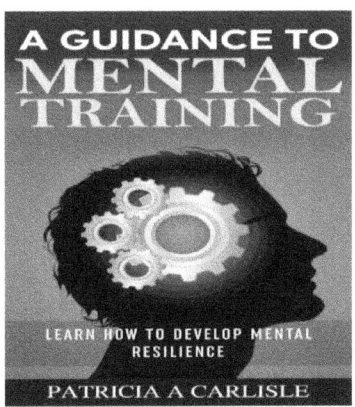

A GUIDANCE TO MENTAL TRAINING: Learn How To Develop Mental

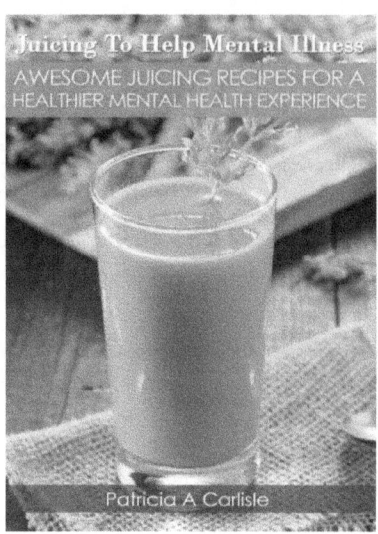

Juicing to Help Mental Illness: Awesome juicing recipes for a healthier mental.

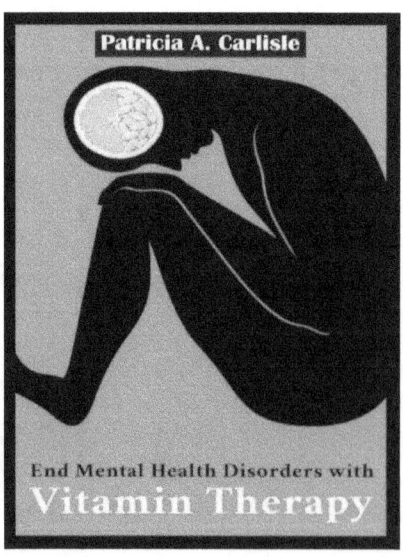

End Mental Disorders with vitamin therapy.

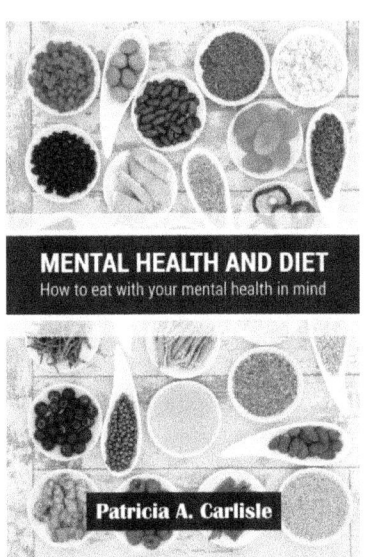

Mental Health and diet: How to eat with your mental health in mind.

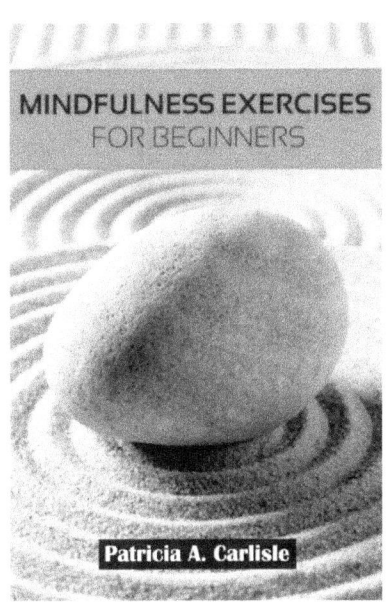

Mindfulness Exercises For Beginners.

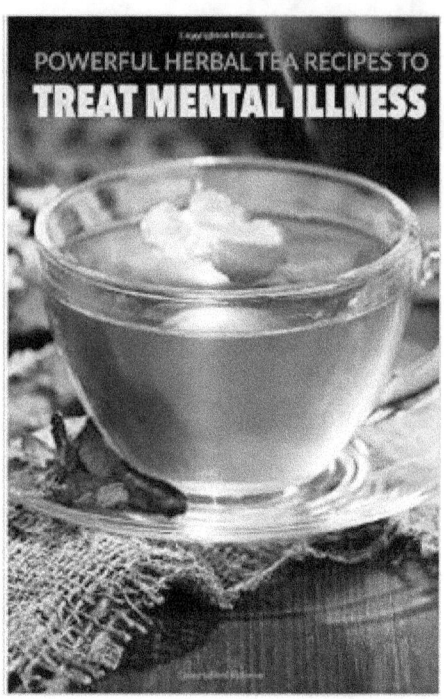

Powerful herbal tea recipes to treat mental illness.

You can simply search for these titles on the Amazon website to find them.

BONUS: SUBSCRIBE TO THE FREE BOOK

Beginners Guide to Yoga & Meditation

"Stressed out? Do You Feel Like The World Is Crashing Down Around You? Want To Take A Vacation That Will Relax Your Mind, Body And Spirit? Well this Easy To Read Step By Step

E-Book Makes It All Possible!"

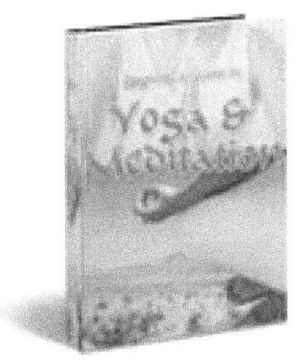

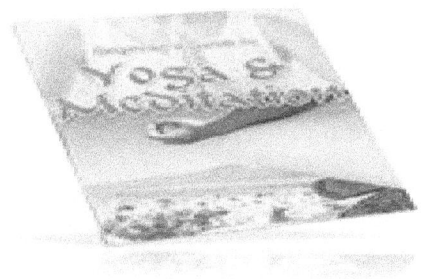

Instructions on how to join our mailing list, and receive a free copy of "Yoga and Meditation" can be found in any of my Kindle eBooks.

NOTES

NOTES

NOTES

NOTES

www.ingramcontent.com/pod-product-compliance
Lightning Source LLC
Chambersburg PA
CBHW070750180526
45168CB00004B/1578